The Business of Makeup Artistry

Toni Thomas

NOTE FROM THE AUTHOR

Becoming a makeup artist is the easy part of your journey, creating your makeup artistry business will be the challenging part. I encourage you to take your time while reading this guide, learn the strategies, implement the new skills you will learn, and follow the business building techniques to execute your makeup artistry business with purpose and intention. You are heading into your new adventure as an entrepreneur, and I am thrilled to see your makeup artistry career grow, the future is going to look beautiful on you!

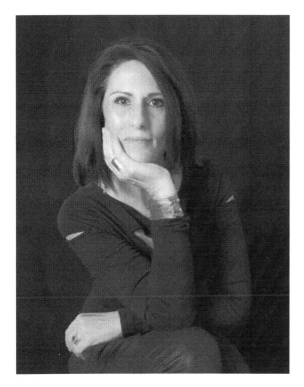

"Makeup artistry is an art, and when used properly it is an art form that creates confidence in those who understand the splendor of it."

I wish you abundant joy & success on your makeup artistry career!

Toni Thomas
Makeup Artist/Author/Educator
Women in Gear: School of Makeup Artistry

Toni Thomas

CONTENTS

ACKNOWLEDGMENTS

This book was a passion for me right from the beginning, and I want to thank everyone who encouraged me to put pen to paper and write down a quick and easy to follow guide for all aspiring makeup artists looking to build their businesses. As we shape our beauty businesses in this ever-changing world of modern technology the process of producing a successful beauty career can be daunting. This book was inspired by my past students who had so many business questions after they completed their makeup courses, it just seemed natural to create a mini-guide as a pathway to help them jump-starting their careers. It is because of you I wrote this guide, and I hope it takes the difficulty out of launching your beauty businesses. It doesn't have to be complicated, but it does require effort, passion, and the determination to stay the course on your new journey.

Toni Thomas

FOREWARD

September 2018, New York Fashion Week, I met and worked with a fantastic makeup artist and team player, Toni Thomas. You know when you meet someone, and you just recognize intuitively that you're going to connect with them? Well, that happened! Toni and I worked a full, fast-paced, productive, 12-hour day; she as a professional makeup artist on my team, and me, the beauty director, overseeing a team of 50 highly skilled and motivated hairstylists and makeup artists.

The beauty business is what I do. It's who I am. I have spent twenty years in this phenomenal industry and for the past fifteen I have owned my own full-service beauty salon, in addition to that, I have worked the past three years as a runway stylist and beauty director in New York City. I have a love and passion for all thing's beauty, makeup, and fashion. My work spans magazines, runway, editorial, pageant, music, tv, and film. In this industry, the possibilities and the extent of your growth are limitless and determined precisely by YOU! In her book, The Business of Makeup Artistry - Your Guide to a Successful Beauty Business, makeup artist, teacher, and author Toni Thomas, tells you exactly how to achieve your beauty industry goals! This informative go-to guide details the eight principles you need to put into practice the skills to not just succeed, but to thrive as a professional makeup artist. She not only teaches on the technical aspect (checklist on how to pack your kit), but she writes and instructs on each of the principles that are guaranteed to set you up for success! Additionally, in this book, you will find websites provided to assist readers further and will direct those who decide to go deeper into researching the topic at hand!

Readers of this book can expect to find instruction on such topics as proper planning and goal setting, brand building, seeing and understanding your desired market and niche, and the importance of marketing and having a great eye-catching logo! Toni also gives honest truths about the competitive, ever-changing, makeup and beauty industry. For example, she explains how looking the part and dressing for success can make the difference between booking a gig or not! She talks about the crucial element of collaboration in our industry, both with other makeup artists, as well as stylists, and often photographers! Also, Ms. Thomas explains how crucial it is in this industry to ALWAYS be punctual and follow through with scheduled appointments!! (NO showing in our industry is a NO NO) These ideas are all extremely beneficial to developing your reputation as a reliable and dependable professional!

Those aspiring to be a professional makeup artist will find this book to be an excellent guide and an invaluable resource! Whether you're new to this industry or a seasoned vet, Toni reminds us of two of the best tools you will need to succeed, Character and Integrity, with a chapter appropriately titled "Build Your Character." I am so pleased that she chose to cover those two topics in her book, trust me when I tell you, these two things will ABSOLUTELY set you apart from the rest! Anybody can have great skill, but add in a phenomenal work ethic, upstanding character, and remarkable integrity... and it's a recipe for success!

The Business of Makeup Artistry takes you on a journey from start to finish. Helpful, informative, uplifting, and motivating. Toni desires long-lasting, successful, lucrative careers for her students and her readers, and reminds us that only YOU have the power to determine precisely how far you will go in your career and journey as a professional makeup artist!

Enjoy the journey!

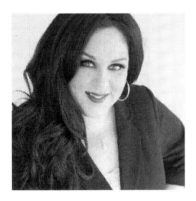

Elizabeth Strong
Master stylist, makeup artist, salon owner.
Beauty director for ASC Magazine NYC.
Email: IG: @estronghair2010

Build Your Foundation

Knowing what your options are in your professional makeup artistry business will help you as you plan your career development and chart a course for your future success. Understanding how to implement your plan will separate you from the average and give you a roadmap to see your future. In this life, we are what we choose to become, and your career options are wide open as a professional makeup artist. A career in makeup artistry has emerged as one of the top professions in the beauty industry and having a robust business strategy will separate you from all the other creatives in the world of professional makeup artistry.

Your Education

The first step in your new career will be to have a solid education in the world of makeup and makeup artistry techniques. There are makeup artistry schools and esthetic schools located all over the world, some are good, some are bad, but most are average. Think positively about your education and remember this is where they teach you the basics of beautification and give you a solid foundation in the field of makeup artistry.

Honestly, it's not where you get your education but what you decide to take from that education that matters the most. I have often heard students complain about the training they have received at a wide variety of schools across the country and my answer to them is always the same, "learn the fundamentals, take what you need, and then improve upon each skill taught by practicing it over and over again until you are proficient." Your education is 50% instruction and 50% what you decide to do with the skills you have learned. It will be up to you to perfect your skills by daily practice and a deep commitment to your craft. To be recognized as the best in the field of makeup artistry, you will need to become the most practiced in your field of study; exercise what you have learned, expand upon it, and never stop learning. Be dedicated enough to enroll in master class workshops throughout your entire career. It is entirely up to you to become the best in your industry.

Maintain Your Credibility

To maintain your credentials as a makeup artist means more than just staying current with the latest trends in makeup it means keeping your credentials or skills current and up to date. The world of makeup artistry is ever changing and it will be up to you to attend continuing education courses offered at your local cosmetology school, vocational school, industry trade shows, or at any makeup artistry event you can find in your area. These classes are designed to keep you in the know of the latest products as well as the latest looks, but the best part of attending a trade show event is building connections with those in your industry who are as passionate about makeup artistry as you.

Practice! It's true the more you practice and develop your skills the more you will increase your level of expertise, and the broader range of skin tones you work with the more you learn to see the skin as your canvas, this will enable you to begin the enhancement of your talents. Having a deeper understanding of skin tones, complexions, and face shapes will assist in your knowledge and education. The more knowledgeable you become, the more opportunities will come your way. Practicing your makeup application skills will build your self-confidence and give you the edge you need to succeed.

Your Niche' Market

To get a closer look at your career options you will first need to understand the who, the what, the when, and the where of your business. To do this, you will need to describe who you are as a makeup artist, such as your skill level and the market you are trying to target. Next, take a look at what your new makeup business does and who it will serve, such as techniques and special skills you possess. You will need to know when you will be open for business, what the hours of your operation are, and where your business is going to be located, this could include a mobile on-location business or a brick and mortar studio. Will you have a local or global market? And, if it's global how far are you willing to travel? Determine what your short and long-term goals are for your business future. Where do you see your business headed in 1 to 3 years and 5 to 10 years? I know this one fact to be true, "if you write your goals down on paper you are seven times more likely to complete them." So get writing and set a plan for your business.

Your Plan

As a makeup artist, it is your job to help your clients look their best for many occasions; you will be doing a wide range of makeup applications for many reasons such as weddings, proms, photo shoots, and other special events. You may even teach makeup by applying makeovers to people who want to update their everyday look. You might specialize in niche markets that assist people in learning how to correct skin issues and cover up defects. As a professional makeup artist is in your best interest to have a solid business plan set in place before you launch your business and begin offering makeup services, look closely at your market area and evaluate your options. If you live in a location with a viable film industry, you may become a makeup artist to film stars or more likely budding film stars by working with on-screen projects. The advantage to this type of makeup business is that you can start working part-time and on a small budget and progress as the demand for your talent increases. As a makeup artist, you'll need the skills and talent to create dramatic effects for people by transforming them with a look they love and it will be up to you to create a solid plan of action to make your business a reality.

If you live in a location that doesn't have a viable film or fashion industry you may want to focus your talents on the wedding industry. In this budding niche' market, you will not only apply makeup to brides and the bridal party, but you will also be teaching skills to your brides and send them home with tips on how to maintain their makeup throughout the wedding day, you might even give them tips to achieve simple and flawless honeymoon makeup. In all instances of your makeup artistry career, you are a teacher, helping your clients learn how to apply and wear the makeup composition that best suits them. Whatever you decide to do with your makeup artistry career you are the only one who can choose the market you want to target. You and only you can determine your skill level and what you are capable of doing. You are the person who is going to create your business plan and set into motion the strategies to make your program a complete success.

Your Dream Board

Having a dream board or online mood board will give you a good idea of the goals you want to achieve with your new business, and it can act as an inspiration to you when your business building gets tough. Trust me when I tell you your business is not always going to be easy. There will be times when you want to throw your hands up in the air and walk away from it all, but having a dream board and a mood board will put your business back into perspective and can allow you to remember why you selected this profession in the first place.

Dream Board

Dream boards are all about vision planning, a place where you determine who you want to be and where you want to go, where you want your career to take you, and the personal and business goals you want to achieve. The best way to get inspired is to write down a few questions for yourself.

What inspires you?

Who inspires you?

Where do you want to go with your career?

What type of looks do you want to create?

Who do you want to work with?

Do you want a studio or on-location business?

If you have a studio what does it look like?

Who would be your dream client?

Do you want to be a runway, fashion, bridal, editorial, or stylized makeup artist?

Your dream board can be created in any format, and you can purchase a simple poster board from any local craft store and start cutting pictures out of magazines or find pictures online to print off. Once you have your images, you can begin to paste those pictures on your board. I suggest you use a "Goals and Outcomes" approach, on the left side apply the photos that meet your business goals, this is where you envision the dream for your business. On the other side of the board use the images that refer to the result of your goals, this is where you might place pictures of a dream makeup case you want to own one day, or the dream car you want to drive, or maybe the dream studio you envision your business to have. The board is made entirely by you, and it should look any way you choose. It is after all your dream board and should encompass your dreams. Don't be afraid to add inspiring quotes to your board or even photos of those makeup artists and their work whom you admire. It is all about creating your idea and the vision of your future and where you see yourself going.

You can also find online places to create your dream

board, check out Pinterest, if you don't already have an account you can generate one and start your business dream board within their site.

Mood Board

Mood boards are an entirely different view of your business, they are the colors and the brand you envision for your business as well as your makeup style. This is where you share the vision you want to show the world of you and your work, this is a good place to start creating your logo. Your mood board will help you create the look for your online portfolio and your website, it is also where you will begin to get an idea of how you want your social media sites to look. The mood board is all about the look and feel of you the artist. Maybe you want to have a bright and vibrant look, or perhaps you are all about soft and subtle. Your mood board is exactly as it sounds, you will be creating the mood for your image, your brand, and how you want others to see you and your work.

Your mood board can be created in a physical or digital format, and most creative artists use mood boards as a tool to illustrate the style they are trying to project of themselves. Your mood board is all about who you are and the projection of your style to others. Your mood board is very important because this is where you will begin to build your brand.

Your Career Options

Here are a few career options for you to consider as you begin to build your career plan and get crystal clear on your vision for your future as a professional makeup artist. On this list are a few career options for you to consider as you move forward in your planning. Your career goals should be an ever evolving plan that grows with you as you grow as an artist. You might start out slow working behind a counter but this can be a be stepping stones to your preferred career goals. No matter what road you travel in your makeup artistry career you need to consider every opportunity presented to you and make career advancement options as you grow in your talents and skill level.

Skincare and Cosmetic Counters

Working the beauty or skincare counter at high-end boutiques or department stores is a good way for you to hone your knowledge and skills. This environment will let you work scheduled hours and may even give you benefits that you may not get working on your own. The cosmetic counters at most retail locations are busy, and you will have the opportunity to meet lots of new people and practice your makeup skills. Many cosmetic counters offer hourly wages and commission on retail sales.

Salon or Day Spa

You can bring your new skills as a makeup artist to a local salon or day spa. Working in a salon may be an option for you but remember in some states in the country a beauty industry license may be required (aesthetician or cosmetologist). The salon environment is a professional setting perfect for a makeup artist, and most salons and spas are very busy with an established clientele that you can pull new clients from. Your job is to market your skills inside the salon and be an interacting part of the environment that you are working in, and the salon management will expect you to create a clientele for yourself and to actively build relationships with the existing clientele. You can do this by creating a flyer or postcard and have monthly specials, then hand them out to customers as they are getting their hair or nails done. Try giving mini-consultations to clients as they are sitting with color or treatments in their hair. You will never find a more captive audience than in a salon where women and men expect the services you provide. Many salons and spas offer hourly wages and commission on retail sales as well as other benefits.

Bridal Makeup Artist

The bridal business has become a billion dollar industry and the wedding day can be one of the most critical days in a woman's life. As a bridal makeup artist, it is your job to enhance the beauty of the bride without changing the way she looks. If you like to travel to different locations and enjoy working in new environments this niche market might be suited for you. It is fast paced and demanding, but the rewards can be huge. Bridal makeup fees can be set very high if you are experienced and willing to travel and if you are doing an entire wedding party, it can be a very lucrative business. Promoting yourself in this market is key to your success, and word of mouth advertising will get you referrals to your business and build a name in this market. This niche market is excellent for a skilled makeup artist.

Theater/Film/Television/HD

Working as a makeup artist in this arena could be challenging. The film and television community is a tight-knit circle, and it's not really what you know but whom you know that can get you through the door. However, once you have proven yourself as a qualified and reliable industry professional this opportunity can prove to be a very lucrative career. The key to entering this arena is to volunteer your services until someone recognizes your talents and brings you into the circle. Film industry makeup artists are never without work. In some cities in the United States, there are makeup artists unions that will put you on their books for call outs. This opportunity is a great way to stay busy and get into other more lucrative jobs.

Fashion Makeup Artist

Many makeup artists aspire to be in the fashion industry to work their craft. The world of fashion requires teamwork, flexibility, creativity, and innovation along with the ability to change direction in a single second. The world of fashion moves at a

breakneck pace and keeping up can be exhausting.
A runway fashion show or a photo shoot can take
days or weeks and sometimes even months to
prepare, but the makeup application must be applied
in a matter of minutes. Backstage can be hectic,
disorganized, or what they like to call controlled
chaos, but if you are willing to work on your feet at a
fast pace and adjust to the whim of a producer,
designer or model this career can be exciting and
glamorous. Usually, the pay is not as good as in the
bridal arena, but if you like the exciting world of
fashion, this might be the career for you. It also
looks excellent on your resume.

Politicians/Business Executives

Makeup Artistry is not just for the fashion industry.
There is a need for makeup artists in many areas but
most certainly in the political as well as the high
powered executive world. These men and women
spend a great deal of time in the public eye on
camera and their need for polished looks are in high
demand, your skills as a makeup artist can help
them to look polished, professional, and well
maintained. When looking at freelance makeup jobs
never leave any stone unturned and take every
opportunity to take the gigs outside of the fashion
industry box. You never know whom you might get
to meet.

Instructor

Becoming a makeup artistry instructor is a rewarding

career that lets you work closely with students who are looking for the same career choice as you. Sharing your love of makeup and of the makeup artistry industry will be your best asset, as well as the ability to relate to many different age groups of students. This career choice will be located in a fun and fast-paced environment where people skills are a requirement not an option. Teaching is rewarding and you will need to not only use your creative side but also your administrative side, creating daily lesson plans, a course curriculum, and testing is all a part of the teaching environment, you will likely be responsible for creating a comprehensive curriculum based on the books and products your school is using. The pay may not be super high but it will be very consistent and may even give you health benefits.

Blogger

Today one of the hottest makeup industry careers is blogging and vlogging (which is video blogging about makeup techniques), and from the rising stars on YouTube, you can see that this industry has taken off like a rocket ship. I suggest you learn the basics of YouTube and creative writing before stepping into this arena, but if you have a good grip on social media and marketing, you could have a very lucrative career in the blogging industry. Take time to learn the inside secrets of social media and implement them in your marketing plan.

Volunteer

Volunteering your services not only looks good on your resume but can also get you the work experience you need and potentially expose your talent to many people. Volunteering at women expos, fundraising events, health fairs and any place where you are visible and meeting people could get you an offer that would advance your career in a new direction.

Dress for success

Every opportunity is a stepping-stone so remember at all times to look your very best, but remember to reflect back to your mood board and project your own personal style. You are the product of what you are trying to sell, and the brand of your work is on your face and in the clothes you choose to wear. Your image is essential when presenting yourself to your clients. People will associate your wardrobe with your skills, this may not be fair, but it is how the world works, so be prepared to create a personal style to go along with your makeup artistry business. Take care to highlight your makeup application by looking polished and not overly made-up. A sophisticated makeup application will outshine an over-done makeup application that looks like it was applied more for the theater than for everyday wear. It is up to you to always be the professional and look the part. If you struggle with how to dress for your new business, try consulting YouTube channels that focus on stylists who dress makeup artists and people who are working in the beauty industry.

The Plan

Your business plan is a working document that will include many documents meant to support your new business, such as a budget, income projections, a mission statement and many more business related goals, remember this document can be updated as you determine what is working and what might not be working for you. One thing is for sure; building your plan is the first step to a solid footing in your new career. The vision for your business has to be crystal clear for you to pursue your dream of becoming a successful makeup artist.

Daily Planner

It is often left out of planning your business but to be successful in this industry you will need to have a handy daily planner to map out your daily goals and to keep your makeup artistry appointments scheduled. Missing an appointment with a client can kill your business instantly. If you are a freelance makeup artist or an on-location makeup artist you need to have a solid schedule to follow and never miss or cancel an appointment. I cannot stress enough how important it is to your career to keep all your appointments. Show up, be prepared and always be the most professional person in the room. This is your business and you are expected to be a professional.

Business Plan Templates

There are thousands of free business plan templates available online. Find one that is simple and to the point and can give you a range of business development tools to help you project your business plan. Don't forget about the financial aspect of your business, you will be responsible for keeping track of your income and expenses and will need to record every penny that comes in and goes out. Find an accountant who can help you do your expense sheets and someone who can help you with end of the year taxes.

Free Financial Tracking

Wave: www.waveapps.com

Free Business Plan Templates

SBA:www.sba.gov/tools/business-plan

SCORE:www.score.org/resources/business-plan-made-easy

Build Your Kit

Building a professional makeup kit separate from your personal kit will take time and money, but it is the number one tool in your business, and you will need to start building your kit immediately. Decide what makeup products you prefer to use on your clients and the products that you can afford to use and then get to work building your pro kit.

When building your pro kit think about the essential products you will need and remember you don't have to use a single line of products or even a professional grade but you do want quality products with easy to use tools and brushes. Consider using a single line of foundation or a pro-grade foundation palette like RCMA. Choosing a single line makes mixing foundations for color matching considerably easier, and it will take up less space when you are toting it around in your on-location makeup travel kit.

Many clients will look at your kit as a reflection of you, and we all know that you are a reflection of your business and your business is what you are trying to build. Your pro kit needs to be professional looking, neat and tidy, and always prepped for any occasion.

Pro Card

Packing your kit can get very costly, but if you are a member of pro artists programs with your favorite cosmetic companies, it can mean huge discounts when you are filling your kit. Pro artist programs are designed to give pro discounts as well as giving you the credibility as a professional makeup artist with that company, and it comes with many perks like product discounts, website listings, makeup workshops, and pro classes for continuing education. You might even get private invites to events where you can hang out with a few celebrities and professional makeup artists. Getting your pro card can be very easy if you take the time to create accounts and submit the required documentation paperwork. Each company varies on the credentials they, but the benefits are enormous and can help you build your pro kit for a hugely discounted rate. Go check out to your favorite makeup company websites, scroll down to the pro artist tab, and follow the guidelines for submission to get your pro card. It can take a bit of effort, but I guarantee it is worth the time you will spend when building your kit.

Pro-Kit Case

Building your kit should be on the top of your list for growing your business and finding the perfect train case or set bag to carry it all in is a critical element. Your makeup case should be easy to haul and have room for all of your products. It should be easy to set up when you arrive at your location and give you an element of sophistication. It should be large enough to hold all of your supplies and have wheels for easy access in and out of the locations you will be going doing makeup. Do your research and spend a little extra on the case itself, after all, you are trying to make your first impression a lasting one.

Packing Your Pro Kit

Here is a list of some essentials you will want in your case:

- Quality Brush Set (Powder Brush, Foundation Brush, Blush Brush, Eye Shadow Crease Blending Brush, Flat Eye Shadow Brush, Liner Brush, Lip Brush)
- Brush Cleaner
- A minimum of four liquid foundations or a pro foundation palette (light, medium, dark; of the same brand so you can mix easily to get the perfect shade)
- Translucent Setting Powder
- Minimum of twenty Eye Shadows (palette form will save you space)
- Blush Colors (peach, pink, plum)
- Lipsticks/Gloss (two nudes, two pinks, two reds, two deep colors)
- Lip Pencils (nude, pink, red, plum)

- Mascara (one lengthening mascara, one waterproof mascara)
- Eyeliners (black/brown/beige)
- Liquid Eyeliner Pen
- Contour/Highlighter Palette
- Concealer Palette
- False Lashes (assorted lengths and sizes)
- Skin Care Products (moisturizer, makeup remover wipes, primer)
- Tools - eyelash curler, lash glue, sponges, spatulas, mixing palette, tweezers, small scissors, mirror, pencil sharpener, disposable tools, small bag for waste.
- Paper Towels
- Hand Sanitizer
- Business Cards
- Client Release Form
- Tall Folding Chair and Portable Makeup Kit Bag (on-location artists)

These are the basics to have in your kit and remember it's better to use quality over quantity. As a new business owner, it can be hard to get the quality you want at a good price so watch for specials and pay attention to what is happening in the market; it will give you clues to get good products at the best prices. You can also research companies that allow you to build your kit at cost effective prices. There are many avenues you can pursue to get your kit filled with the products you want and love. Try becoming an affiliate for your favorite products or become a distributor for a direct sales line of cosmetics that can give you a second avenue of income in the form of commissions.

Supplemental Income

You are not a smart businessperson if you are not earning a commission or income from some of the products you use on your clients. You should always be making product recommendations for your clients as you are applying their makeup and certainly on products they love, I can guarantee they will be asking your opinion on what to use and where they can get the products you are using. If you plan to have a great business, you need to be able to market and sell a few products that you love and use in your pro kit.

Remember your kit is a reflection of you and therefore is the soul of your business, as such, it requires you to pack it in a fashion that is efficient, effective and gives you the creative energy you need to be the best in your business.

Makeup Train Cases and Supply Companies

www.zuca.com

www.glamcor.com

www.shanycosmetics.com

www.thepromakeupshop.com

Build Your Portfolio

As far as your business goes building your portfolio is one of the essential elements for your success as a freelance makeup artist. Creating your portfolio is not only critical, but expected in today's world of photo-driven social media marketing. Clients no longer accept that you are the best in your profession; they want to see that you are the best and they want to know that you have taken the time to create a look-book for them to review.

Your portfolio must contain your top work and have the ability to showcase your talents in many ways. If you are a well-rounded makeup artist, you may need to have more than one look-book. If you are working as a bridal makeup artist, your potential clients will want to check out your bridal looks. You may have prom girls who want to see your work and their mothers may want to see that your looks fit the age group of these young women. You might also need a look-book for the everyday woman looking for a makeover session and makeup lessons. Don't forget about your specialty and portrait makeup looks these will need to be showcased as well. You can see where this is going, and it means that if I am your customer, I don't want to slog through hundreds of pictures looking for the makeup application I want to achieve. I expect you the professional to have it created and have it organized into categories so I can easily access and find the look I want.

Creating Your portfolio

In today's market you no longer carry around a physical portfolio book with your makeup looks inside; instead, you are pulling out your smartphone or tablet to share your online portfolio, Instagram can be a great portfolio site if you only post your makeup work. A website or Facebook business page is often the easiest way to send your potential clients a link to your portfolio before you ever meet them in person. In today's technology-based world it will be expected that you have an online portfolio filled with your work that it is relevant to the look they are trying to achieve.

Building your online portfolio will require more than just your image gallery; it will also be the place where you house your online resume and your online biography with a current photograph of you. Even if you are starting your makeup artistry career, you will need to create your online bio. Your bio should contain some key facts about yourself such as your education and your certified skill level or whether you are a self-taught well-seasoned makeup artist. It should also provide a brief background on you and your interests. Make it fun and exciting with just a touch of personal info. Talking about your own life is acceptable to a point, but it should only be the professional details about you and your profession along with any relevant information such as competitions you have entered, any fashion shows you worked, any awards you have received and any volunteer work that directly relates to your career.

Your Photography

You are in charge of capturing your portfolio images, and in so doing you will need to make sure to photograph every one of your practice models as well as your paying customers, this will require a good quality camera or a smartphone that lets you generate quality pictures. I recommend taking a short class on photography to learn how to use your camera or your phone to capture the best photos possible. There are some great photo apps you can use to edit your photo for better quality and color. If you are on a budget, then utilize YouTube to watch free videos on capturing and editing your photos for your online look-book. I also recommend using an excellent online photo editor to edit and size your pictures to give them a polished look. Check out canva.com, which is an excellent photo-editing site

Professional Photography

Don't forget if you are working in an environment where a professional photographer will be taking photos that you need to exchange business cards and ask that any images of the clients be shared with you for your business portfolio. They may be happy to share their photos as long as you credit their work with each photo you use and send business their way, this is a win-win scenario for both you and the photographer, you get high-quality pictures, and they get exposure to your online presence. You might also try to bring in a professional photographer for stylized events you are working on, this is a great time to offer to trade services in exchange for their high-quality photos. You might have to pay for their time to be there, but you may be able to get some incredible images to use in your portfolio. It is never beneath you to try and negotiate with your fellow professionals, we are all in the business of marketing ourselves so try and give something of value in exchange for something of value.

Release Forms

You are also in charge of making sure that each person you photograph will allow you to use his or her image in your portfolio. I recommend that you carry release forms for every person who may get their photo taken during your makeup session. If your client agrees to let you use their image, it can be used for your online business page and will not cause any legal problems for you in the future. It is your responsibility to treat your business as a legal entity and to take all the precautions that any professional would.

Time is Money

You are a professional makeup artist and a businessperson, and your time is valuable, it will be up to you to always charge rates that are comparable to your skills. Do not let others devalue your work by negotiating you into a price rate that doesn't make business sense. You are a professional makeup artist, and your skills are needed and wanted by many, stick to your listed prices and do not negotiate terms that leave you feeling devalued. Your self-confidence will guide you in the process of charging the rates you know are worth your time, so be proactive and always check in with fellow makeup artists to gage price comparable. Don't let the "best friend" discount put you in the "best friend" poor house, your time is valuable, and you have overhead costs just like any other professional, your skills demand to be rewarded just like any other professional business person.

Accepting Payment

Speaking of money, now would be a good time to discuss how you will be accepting payment for your services and the best way to take payments in the world of freelance makeup artistry. I suggest you start by having a contract written up in a word document that you can send to potential clients by email. This binds you and your client to an agreement of financial payment for services rendered. If you are doing large events where you are doing makeup on two or more people it is wise to get at least a 50% deposit prior to the event that will make their event a booking on your calendar. This protects you against last minute cancellations.

There are many ways to accept payment, you can utilize PayPal, Point of Sale with Square Card Reader, or create an online booking app attached to your portfolio website that can handle a payment transaction when a client books for your services. Remember a contract is binding and if you accept any deposits for your services you must never cancel with your scheduled client.

Social Media Portfolio Sites

Social media has come leaps and bounds in the past couple of years, and there are so many social media sites to choose from it can get overwhelming, but if you stick to your goal of business first, you can narrow down your choices. Think of your social media business sites as a storefront that showcases all your best makeup looks in the storefront window. If we owned a store, we wouldn't post pictures of our kids, our dogs, or a series of self portraits of you at a party on the window; we would put up photos of our best work trying to attract our optimal client. Your social media business sites are your storefront.

What sites are best for promoting and engaging customers? There are many to choose from, here is a list of a few social media sites you can use as business pages for showcasing your work.

Facebook Business Page: facebook.com
Instagram: instagram.com
Pinterest: pinterest.com
Google Business Page: google.com

Online Portfolio Sites

Portfolio sites are online sites to upload your makeup work and can be photo sites or one-page websites that host your online portfolio. You don't need to hire a web designer in today's world click on the host sites and most if not all have templates to choose from and all you need to do is upload your work and a bio about yourself. Some online sites are more advanced than others, and some offer more than one tab to provide you with options other than just your photos. Some sites will have tabs for your services, for your photos, for your bio, and for your social links. It will be entirely up to you where you choose to house your online portfolio but having one is crucial to your business. Below are a few places you can go and check out their offerings for online websites and online portfolio collections.

www.wix.com

www.bigblackbag.com

www.foliosnap.com

www.viewbook.com

Build Your Character

I would be remiss if I skipped over a topic not many people like to discuss. The character of a person determines that which generates their success. We build our character over time and through the lessons we learn in life, not everyone chooses to go in a positive direction, and not everyone understands the value of having a good character. So what does having a good character have to do with your makeup business? In my opinion, it has everything to do with your business and your future success. Good character is a reflection of good personality traits, and you, as a professional makeup artist will need to encompass a vast majority of these traits.

Good Character

The dictionary defines character as "the mental and moral qualities distinctive to an individual."

Abraham Lincoln said, "Reputation is the shadow. Character is the tree." Having a strong character is doing the right thing because it is the right thing to do.

Good character means a solid foundation and an understanding of who you are and what your value system is. It encompasses a strong work ethic followed by living your life in a standard that reflects positively on you and others. It is the foundation of choosing to be inherently good by nature even when it is easier to do otherwise. It is, in fact, a reflection of the choices we make in the hard parts of our lives that bring about positive results in our future. Each of us has the ability to live our life with a good and strong character, and the result of your decision to live your life with good character will be lasting relationships that are built on trust.

Discretion

As a working professional in the beauty and makeup industry working closely with others is a huge part of your job, this means often you will hear things that others say to co-workers and other people in a salon or studio setting. You will be told things you may not want to know, and you will be trusted with knowledge given freely to you by clients and customers. I have found in this industry that when working closely with our clients, they tend to trust you with some of their intimate life details. It is not your place to repeat their stories nor for you to judge their person based on the things they tell you. When working so closely with others while in such close proximity it is a distinction of your character to hold true to your values and stay focused on the job at hand. You are the first and last stop in the transfer of information.

In your working profession you may come into contact with a wide variety of personalities, and at times not every one of those individuals will be looking out for you and your best interest. It is up to you to protect your good character by only taking jobs that feel right to you. That being said, I am trying to tell you that your career is earned through mutual trust and respect. Do unto others, as you would have them do unto you, act professionally at all times and keep discretion close to your business model, this will bring you a great deal of respect in your career not only by your peers but by your clients as well.

Beauty Professional Code of Conduct and Ethics

It is easy to gain an understanding of your career field code of ethics, it was written and laid out for you by the beauty professional code of conduct and ethics committee. You can access this @ www.beautycouncil.ca

Build Your Network

Building relationships will prove to be your greatest asset as you venture out into your new business and the power of attraction marketing can skyrocket your business.

In truth, the best part of your new career will be all the amazing relationships you get to make. The law of attraction says, "that you attract into your life whatever you think about." It is in these thoughts that we create our realities. Success can be thought, but the action is required to make this thought a truth. These thoughts and actions have to have specific positive outcomes to be considered success. What you do with your thoughts will inherently lead you in the direction you are trying to go in. So think positive thoughts and be successful in your business!

Leave Your Comfort Zone

To be successful in your new makeup artistry business, you will need to add two skills; self-confidence and the ability to leave your comfort zone. The ability to step out into the world of building relationships and make real connections with others by sharing your passion with them while appreciating their passions in life is your number one objective. Living out loud and in your own truth is hard in a world that can be so critical of others. But remember if it was easy anyone could do it! And trust me when I tell you it will not be easy. However you are stronger than you think, you are brave and can overcome all hardships by applying a straightforward rule. Live your life as a fearless queen!

True Connection

Reaching into the hearts of others to make real connections will require a personal connection to people you do not know. Here is the truth, "to be a success and get to the top you will need to do that which 99% of the population is not willing to do!" Imagine that you are in the top 1% of the people around you; it is your chance to project your self-confidence in your skills as a makeup artist and a person who is capable of whatever comes your way.

Building relationships is a skill set that needs to be practiced daily just like you need to practice your makeup techniques daily. It may come easily to you to make friends, and it may be second nature for you to reach out and touch someone's life and appreciate others. It may even be easy for you to pick up the phone and circumvent today's technology-based connections and make a personal connection. If this is easy for you to do, then I would say you are well on your way to success, because building relationships will be a skill you are going to need to be the best in your industry.

Be Fearless

To have a successful makeup artistry career takes courage and a fearless approach to life and your profession. You will be the risk taker of the bunch, the one who leads the way in the industry and who takes the chances no one else is willing to do. You will need to learn how to appreciate others and learn to connect on a more personal level, and this will require good glad-handing, genuinely getting to know people and taking the time to learn about what others want and need. You are in the business of creating value for others and showing them the benefits of your business.

Relationships

Never underestimate the power of you. You are and always will be the figurehead of your new business so be genuine and always be true to you. The power of self can carry its weight in gold and will give you the courage to continue in your new business even when it's hard, and it's going to be hard. It will be up to you to market yourself, build your clientele and build the relationships that will continue to open up new opportunities. Relationship building means making genuine connections and then following up and following through with your new friendships.

If you are looking to work in the theater as a professional makeup artist, it will be up to you to find local theater groups to join on Facebook and make connections with people who are currently working they craft in this arena. You can also walk into any theater company and offer your services. If you want to be a runway makeup artist you will need to reach out to runway fashion producers and engage with them about the skills you have to offer, send them your portfolio link and ask if you might get an invitation to their next show. If you want to work as an editorial makeup artist then it's time to start connecting with photographers who are currently submitting their work and let them know of your desire to collaborate.

Collaboration

Collaboration is key to your makeup artistry success. No matter how many times I say it in this book, you need to be connecting with those individuals who are currently working in your desired industry and build relationships. You are the only one who can achieve your goals, and you are the only one who can make them become a reality. Collaborating is the perfect way for everyone to reach a common goal. Photographers love makeup artists because we can make their hours of editing substantially smaller while they work on perfecting the feel for the editorial submissions. Theaters are always in need of makeup artists. Wedding planners are always looking for makeup artists to refer to their clients. Hairstylists love working with makeup artists during the wedding season, these stylists are inundated by bridal parties and need a makeup artist to complete the look a bride and her bridal party want. The list of collaborations for makeup artists is endless, it all depends on what your goals are and what area of the industry you want your career as a makeup artist to take you.

Build Your Value

As a beauty industry professional one of the most challenging tasks is determining your value and worth, but this can easily be accomplished by doing your research and due diligence. You can start your research by going online to aw website called o*net online at www.onetonline.org to see what others are earning in the beauty industry across the United States. As of the date of publishing for this book, O*net says, "that the median wages for makeup artists in the US is $21.30 per hour or $44,310 per year." Not too shabby for a professional freelance makeup artist in the beauty industry and it can be achieved if you apply yourself to your profession and take the time to build your skill level and create a professional business.

Monetary Determination

You and only you can determine your monetary value. You build up your worth as you build up your skills and your professional presence. Time is money as we have already discussed, so you want to be very careful not to devalue your skills by not charging appropriately for your services and time. You can easily do this by doing your homework and research.

What are others charging for their services? What scale are others using to determine their worth and how can you become a viable asset in the industry?

There are stages to building your value and determining your monetary worth. Try to look at the big picture, not the short-term quick fix. If this is your business and your long-term career goals are to become a full-time beauty industry professional then building your business will start by working in your career field as much and as often as possible. You must be working and practicing your craft every day if you are not doing hands-on makeup applications daily, then you need to stay in the know by researching and reading. Follow all the professionals who are making it happen in the world of makeup artistry. Stay connected to the fashion and beauty industry and follow all the current trends. Determine what trends are lasting and what trends are coming. It is up to you to create the professional world you want to be a part of and to determine your value and worth for your time and services.

Gaining Your Value

The first step is getting your feet wet, or more likely

getting familiar with how this industry works. It is a time of building your network, practicing your skills and gaining confidence in your abilities, and this is where you practice your craft every day and start building your business acumen. You are beginning to get a feel for your professional surroundings and learning how to assert your monetary value. You are developing your plan, your presence, and your knowledge to gain a reputable and dependable presence in the makeup artistry industry. This stage is your 1 to 3-year phase and will require you to be well prepared for every person who will try and get more for less. It is also the period in your career that will require you to be a sensible and robust business professional and have a flexible backbone. It will require you to overcome any doubts about what to charge for your services, and it is when you will do your research and determine your worth. It is the period in your business when you will practice your skills each and every day and obtain as much knowledge about the makeup artistry industry as possible. It is the convenient time for you to volunteer your time and services, attend as many professional meetings as possible and create a buzz about your new business. You will be the person who will share your enthusiasm with others and get the media talking about you. You are the professional so to be on your game and be the best.

Unleashing Your Power

The second step in your career is to ascertain your value through research and study. You are the only one who can create value in your business, and it is worth your time to create a monetary value that is above reproach. As a true professional freelance makeup artist, your time is valuable. If you are traveling to clients your time is even more valuable and the costs associated with this need to be considered. You need to have an income that substantiates your true professionalism and when others tell you they can get the same services elsewhere for a better price it is your responsibility to remind them that you and your services are worth the prices you are advertising.

Why? Because they are getting you and you know your value, and you need to translate to them how valuable you are.

How? Direct them to all your social sites, show them your look book, get them the link to your website reviews, and always be a professional in every aspect of your interactions with others.

Do not devalue yourself to fit into the mass mold. Take the time to get a good understanding of your value and how valuable the services are that you provide, share the results of your work that you have put out in the world and what you expect for monetary value in return. You are the business professional and will be expected to maintain a high level of business wisdom.

It is up to you to create the value of the industry you are working in and never let others take away your credibility. You have worked hard to master your craft, and you need to ascertain what you are willing to negotiate at the time you begin your negotiations. Do not let what others charge for their services be the deciding factor in what you charge for yours. The rule of thumb in this industry is for every one hundred faces you apply makeup to you have added an extra layer of value to your services and their monetary value.

Building your value will be difficult, most of us tend to think of our skills as less than worthy and find it hard to promote ourselves to others. It is our instinct to admire those we believe are more talented or influential than ourselves. When you are building your value, it is the time to be brave and acknowledge your skills are valuable and in high demand. As you start to develop your value, you should adhere to the principle of daily practice to keep our skills honed to perfection while exploring every artistic opportunity that comes your way. As you build your value, you will also begin to create your brand, and as you build your brand, you must start to look at who you are and what you want to represent. How will you promote your value and brand to others? Now is the time to unleash the power of you.

Talent and Value

Talent means nothing without consistent effort and practice, or in general terms hard work. To be successful in your makeup artistry career you must surround yourself with those who work hard, have the same goals, and who make you look better than you are. It will be up to you to use each day as an opportunity to improve, to be better, to get a little bit closer to your career dreams and goals. It might sound like a lot of work, but the more you accomplish, the more you'll want to do, the higher you'll want to reach. As long as you have the hunger for success, you will always have the power within you to achieve it. You bring the value of your talents to others, and in so doing you will be the person whom others will turn to when they are looking for your particular skill set.

Consistency is Key

We often hear these words but what do they mean for you the artist? Consistency is merely doing the same thing over and over again until it becomes an everyday part of your life and second nature to what you do each day. A painter who is successful paints every day, they are drawn to the canvas like a moth to a flame, they are unable to resist the yearning to paint. The same holds for you, the makeup artist, the mediums may be different but to be recognized as the best you must be consistently working your craft every day and share your work so others can see your talent. Being persistent in your art and sharing your work for others to see will be the most important aspect of your career. It might mean giving makeup tips regularly, so you are helping others solve their problems or showcasing your work so others know how talented you really are. No matter how you market your talent and skill, you will need to be consistent in your effort and persistent with those who you reach out to every day to collaborate with. As I have said before, "collaboration is the key ingredient to your success as an artist and an influencer."

Take the time to build your value as a makeup artist and build the relationships that will lead you to amazing collaborations with other talented people.

Build Your Brand

Creating your professional brand will take time and patience, but it will be the recognition of you and your brand that defines you as a professional. Your top of mind awareness will determine your success as a makeup artist, and it will be up to you to create a brand that shows your true self, a you that embodies your passion in a fun and professional way, while at the same time giving you an edge over your competition. It will be up to you to keep your brand in the spotlight and to provide it with the look and feel you want to project.

Why create a brand? What will it accomplish and how does it help you get an edge up on your career?

Your brand will keep a connection between your profession and your person; it will be the factor that binds you and your skills with you the artist. Think of all the professional makeup artists whom you follow or admire? I would wager that just speaking their first name you know exactly what their brand is and who someone might be talking about. You might even know who a makeup artist is based solely on only their logo and what they do better than anyone else in the industry. You might even know what their signature look is. Maybe even a symbol will conjure up images of their face or one of their makeup applications.

What about an application or makeup look, could you link it to one of your favorite makeup artists? If so, then this is called a personal brand, sight recognition that brings you back to the name and face of a person.

How do you begin to create your professional brand?

First, you must take a very close look at how others see you right now and then determine how you want others to see you as you move forward with your career and your brand. Think about your favorite makeup artist you might follow on Instagram or on YouTube, what are they doing that keeps you coming back for more? What sets them apart from their competitors? What gives them their huge fan base and what gives them their own special brand?

They have taken the time and given the effort to create a look and a brand that sets them apart and gives them influence. They may or may not be more talented than any other makeup artist but they have stuck to the credo of consistency and persistence with their brand and their market. The same will be required of you as you start to plan out your marketing and your professional branding. Take the time to answer questions about yourself and keep them close to you as you set about creating your professional brand.

1. What reminds people of you?
2. What are friends and family tagging you in on social media?
3. What are others saying about you and your work?
4. What are you passionate about that you can bring to your work?
5. What are five items you think of when you think of yourself?
6. What are three things others think of when they think of you?
7. What is one symbol you can quickly relate too?
8. What makeup application is your signature look?
9. What separates you from other makeup artists
10. What inspires you??

To determine your professional brand, you need to start a list and get others involved. Write down how you perceive yourself and your style of artistry. Then ask others how they see you and your form of makeup artistry. Then start to get more specific; what can you incorporate into your world and professional self that will create your brand.

Logo

Your logo will be a massive part of your brand, when deciding what logo you want and how it should look, make sure it is a reflection of you and how you want others to see you. Make it original and easy to read. Give it colors that stand out and use a font that is bold yet creative. Be original and be you and be specific about your niche' market. The more specific you are, the better your services will be received.

Business Cards

Your business card should have your logo as well as your name, phone number, website, and online portfolio or online look-book. Make it easy to read with fonts that are true to you and your brand. I always tell my students to create a look that is fun, original to them and gives precisely the idea of how they want others to see them.

Online

Your online presence such as your website, your makeup portfolio, and your social media sites all need to look and feel similar to have a strong brand in this industry. They will need to have a consistent color scheme and images that people associate with you and your brand. Spend the time creating mood boards for yourself and establish a look and feel that you can relate too. Develop a plan for your brand and give it depth by adhering to the rules of brand building (simplicity, consistency, and ease) these three factors will determine your online presence and will start to accelerate your professional brand hitting the target for your intended market. It will define who you are professionally and will give you the credibility in your makeup artistry career. Don't worry if you have an online presence now that isn't working, take the time to review your sites and update them to reflect your new brand and the image you want to project.

Videos

Building your brand through videos can be one of the fastest ways to get your professional brand out to the world. Be creative and fun but more importantly, it is in your best interest to be consistent. It will be up to you to be unique, funny, original, and inspiring. One fact to think about with videos, 78% of all videos get 8 seconds of run time, but if a video is made well, they are watched through to the end. The first rule of videos, you only have 8.25 seconds to grab the attention of your audience, so it will be up to you to start your video with a great intro.

Building your brand is more than a logo, it is also you, and how you present your image to others. A professional brand will encompass the complete package that is you, the makeup artist. It will be up to you to create healthy relationships, build credibility, and trust in your industry. One of the most critical aspects of your brand will be to create a professional trust with others who know you are ethical, reliable and rock solid in your makeup skills. You will need to stay well connected to your brand as a consistent part of your everyday life.

Author Your Career

You are the author of your career, so write the book that others want to read and make it so valuable that they can't imagine their lives without your daily inspiration. Authoring your makeup artistry career and your professional brand will take time, effort and a daily routine that will require you to step out of your comfort zone and into the unknown every day.

Build Your Influence

It takes time and effort to build up your influence in any industry but most especially in the beauty industry. Even after almost thirty years in this industry half of which was teaching students in both skill and business building I still have to keep working the skills I have mapped out in this book to stay current as an expert in my field. To be an influencer you need to have a solid base of followers or clients who believe in the knowledge you have to share with them. To be an influencer means others will look at you as a specialist in your field, and they will be inclined to follow your direction and will pass on your information to others.

How do you become an influencer in your makeup artistry career?

You must be engaged with your audience and have the ability to make them feel as if you are talking directly to them and taking them on a visual journey that inspires them. Influence is a gift that very few people know how to acquire in this industry. There are however a few ways to build up the skills necessary to become an industry influencer.

Become an Influencer

To be an influencer you start by mastering all of the previous skills in this book and then you take your career to the next level. You up your game by pushing yourself farther from your comfort zone than you have ever been before and you start connecting with those in the industry who are going to help you rise to the top. Rising to the top requires you to put forth an added level of effort. One of the first things you can do is join your local beauty industry association or union. Get involved in their meetings and events, connect with people at those meetings who will ask you to present yourself as an industry leader. Do your homework and find out how you can help them fill in gaps at events and help them teach others in the industry to solve problems. Helping others solve their problems is the way to present yourself as an industry leader. Attend the beauty industry association events nationwide and enroll in their courses or their competitions, next thing you know you could be leading one of their workshops or sitting on the judge's panel of a national competition. It's entirely up to you how much you get involved but take the time to get involved and make an impact.

Article Submissions

To become an influencer you might want to start writing articles for online publications or hard copy magazines. Find a topic you know is trending in the industry and put your spin or view on it. Write up the article and start submitting it for publication. Most beauty publications are always looking for experts in the field to write articles or get quotes from industry insiders who are on the ground working in the trade. You have the expertise, you know what you want to say, now is the time to say it and get your thoughts out to the public and influence the beauty industry in your own unique way.

Editorial Publication

As a working makeup artist who wants to be an influencer, you need to work with photographers who are willing to make submissions for publication. As the makeup artist will get credit and your work could be seen by millions of readers. This is the perfect time to create a signature look you have developed and get it out to the masses. Once you have created a look that is trending you will be an influencer in your industry.

Getting your work published in any editorial magazine or online publication will boost your influence in this industry. You are the only one who can make this happen and to do this you will need to build long and lasting relationships with editors, photographers, stylists and those who submit editorial work.

Public Speaking

One of the best ways to be an industry influencer is to be an invited or paid guest speaker at local and national events. This will build your following quicker than any other type of work you do. As a guest speaker you become the expert on the topic you are discussing and will be recognized as an industry leader. Do your homework and know your topic. Publish articles or a book on your chosen subject and then start submitting your name to events where they need subject matter experts to speak.

The trick to public speaking is to have a well thought out subject matter and the ability to share your topic on a personal level with your audience. Help others overcome their challenges and solve their most pressing matters.

You will also need to have the ability to stand up in front of large crowds and be funny and informative. This would not be the time to wing it, speaking at conferences and events requires a well-prepared speaker who can handle direct questions and take the pressure of speaking in front of hundreds of attendees.

Invited Guest

Try to become an invited guest to a beauty event in your area. This might mean you sit on an open panel discussion with other influencers or to a local or national talk show where you are the expert sharing your knowledge. As an invited guest you will be discussing topics that relate to listeners who are looking to you as the expert. Be prepared to answer any questions that may or may not be related to the subject matter. This is the time to be thoughtful and insightful.

Brand Ambassador

Influencers are also brand ambassadors for other companies. This usually happens when you begin to build large followings on your social media sites and your work and knowledge begins to get recognition. Stay true to your image and your brand when you become an ambassador for other companies. Do they fit into your audience following and do you believe in the products or services you as representing?

As an influencer, you will need to refer to your own personal code of ethics. Others will be watching you very closely and following your lead, take it upon yourself to be the leader of what you professional believe in and stick to your fundamental roots.

To become a professional makeup artist, it takes more than a train case and a set of good brushes, it takes hard work, a well-established plan, and the desire to be the best in your industry.

To be successful, you must surround yourself with

those who work hard, smile easy, and who make you look better than you really are, those who support you and your work. Use each day as an opportunity to improve, to be better, and get a little closer to your goals and dreams. It might sound like becoming a success in this industry takes a lot of work, but the more you accomplish, the more you will aspire, and the higher you will go in your makeup artistry career. As long as you have the hunger for success, you will always have the power within you to achieve it. To be the best you must be a part of something bigger than yourself.

I wish you abundant joy and success in your makeup artistry career.

ABOUT THE AUTHOR

Opening her first brick and mortar salon in 1993 Toni Thomas was a mere twenty-nine years old when she began her first venture into the world of business and beauty. Jumping in with both feet has always been her style and remains her style today. Her career has revolved around the beauty industry and sharing her passion for beauty business success is what she has come to love.

Teaching makeup artistry, entrepreneurship, and business to those who are willing to take a leap of faith on themselves is what she aspires to do the rest of her life. She is the founder of Women in Gear: School of Makeup Artistry an online education portal for aspiring makeup artists. She is an industry leader in business building across for the beauty and teaching business building skills is one of her favorite topics.

Born and raised in a small town in Montana, she moved to the Washington DC area with her executive husband and now travels extensively between her home in the mountains of Montana and her home by a lake in Virginia, she travels to New York City as an invited runway makeup artist for New York Fashion Week and is a full time working makeup artist.

She believes no matter how good you think you are, there is always a better version of your talent to be developed, so take the time to practice your skills every day and always say yes to every opportunity that comes your way.

You can follow her

Instagram: @toni_thomas_mua

Facebook: @tonithomasmua

Made in the USA
Middletown, DE
02 September 2019